victoria davis

Shakti

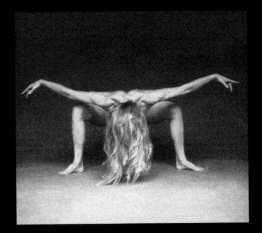

Foreword

What I love about the process and path of yoga is that the compass is directed towards our core self - our flowing essence - who we are when all of the coverings fall away. Being naked is a spiritual metaphor of our original state for it is how we arrived in the world through our mother's loins and were celebrated for the first time. Lalla, the beloved 14th century yogini from Kasmir, literally lived in a state of naked awareness with only her long, dark hair for her robes. She is known for her poetic teachings, which she spread through her ecstatic song and dance, such as this song below:

The soul, like the mooni
is new and always new again
and I have seen the ocean
continuously creating.

Since I washed my mind
and my body, I too,
am new, each moment new.

My teacher told me one thing
Live in the soul.

When that was so,
I began to go naked and dance.

Lalla celebrated living the reality of our essential oneness, which she often described as "Shiva and Shakti making love in the jasmine garden". Within yoga, Shivashakti are the One whose embrace brings about the many. Shiva is the seed of consciousness, the male principle. Shakti is the feminine force, which manifests consciousness, the energy that animates form. Thus, Shakti is this book that you are holding, these word symbols, the breath moving us, the sounds in the background, the chair that is cradling you, the earth that we are rooted upon. As "Shaktima" - the great mother - she is our body, the light in every cell, the food, breath, water, love, intelligence that sustains us. Shakti is the creative force that transcends gender but is celebrated through the feminine form for her life-giving power.

Victoria's images celebrate Shakti through the yogini - women whose bodies - like Lalla - have become their temple, their source of discovery and renewal, the place of re-membering our life force. Here you see the many aspects of the feminine force - strong as a live oak, fluid as the sea, soft and still as the fertile earth, changing like the moon - sister, daughter, mother, lover, leader, dancer. In a time, when so many women feel a need to "fix" their form externally, the yogini embraces shakti with love and radiates that communion from the inside out.

The opportunity to play with Victoria was healing for everyone involved for it was a chance to not be bound by external perfection but to allow the pranashakti to find her spontaneous, naked dance. Victoria as a yogini herself knows how to look for natural essence and bring her to light. In yoga, this is referred to as darshan, "seeing the Divine". May these images remind of us of our flowing spirit, of the innate power and grace of our lifeforce, of our inherent freedom that yoga serves.

Jai Shaktidevi!
Victory to the Shining One!

Namaste
Shiva Rea

Acknowledgements

Where do I begin? It all started with my girlfriend Raquel...who pushed me onto my path as a photographer. Then Alison....who walked me into my first yoga class. My journey took the most beautiful turn....and this book was born. First I must thank all of my models....you are the inspiration behind this project...and I am grateful. Thank you to all of my friends.....for your never-ending support. Shiva and Leah...for your beautiful words. John Casey, for translating all of the sanskrit. Russ, we couldn't have done this without you. Thank You. Clint, for your enthusiasm and guidance. Amy. You are amazing. What would I do without you. My daughter, Savannah...thank you for your patience. You are my angel. And of course, my parents. Thank you for always believing in me. You have given me the wings to fly.

Models

Leah Alperin, Micheline Berry, Rosalind Brown, Kristin DiGaetano
Anne Greene, Terra Gold, Rebekah Henty, Hala Khouri, Stephanie Layne
Noelle Maremont, Alison McLea, Malachi Melville, Shiva Rea
Miriam Rothman, Joeanna Sayler, and Erika Schnicke

follow your heart...

for twyla

photographs

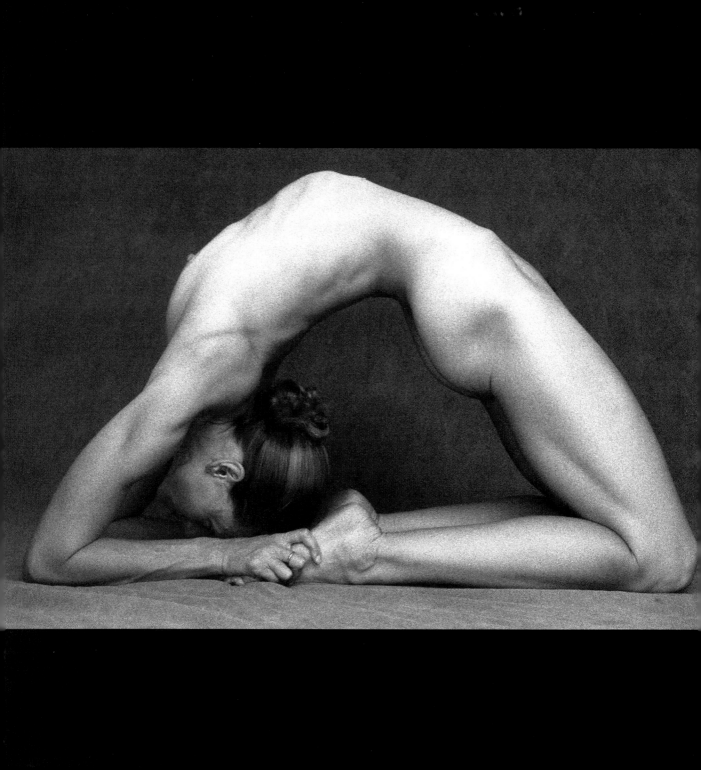

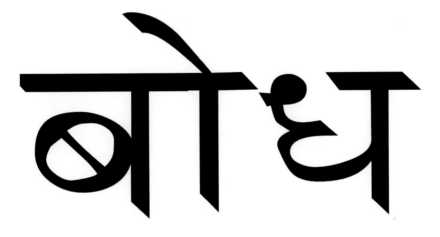

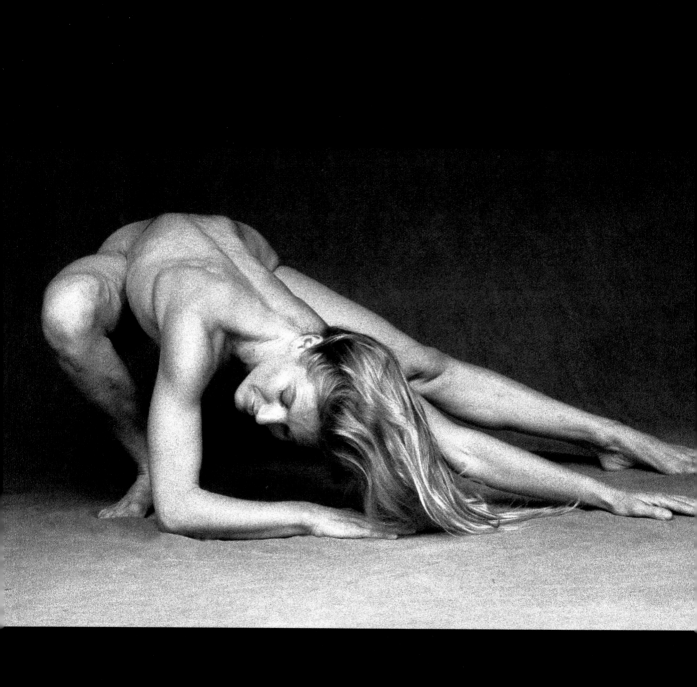

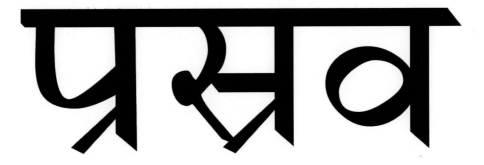

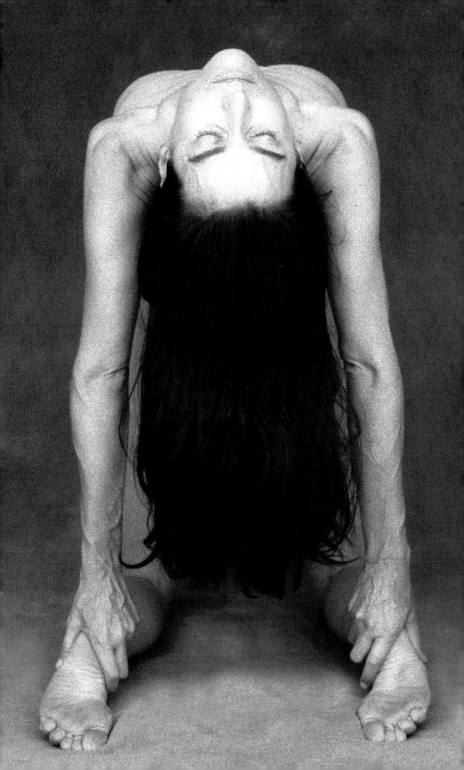

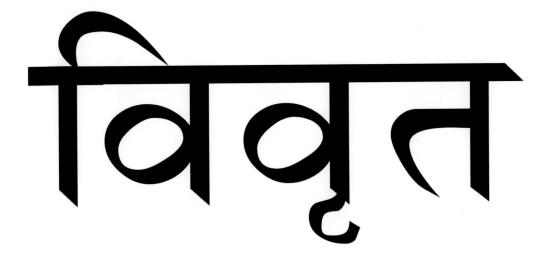

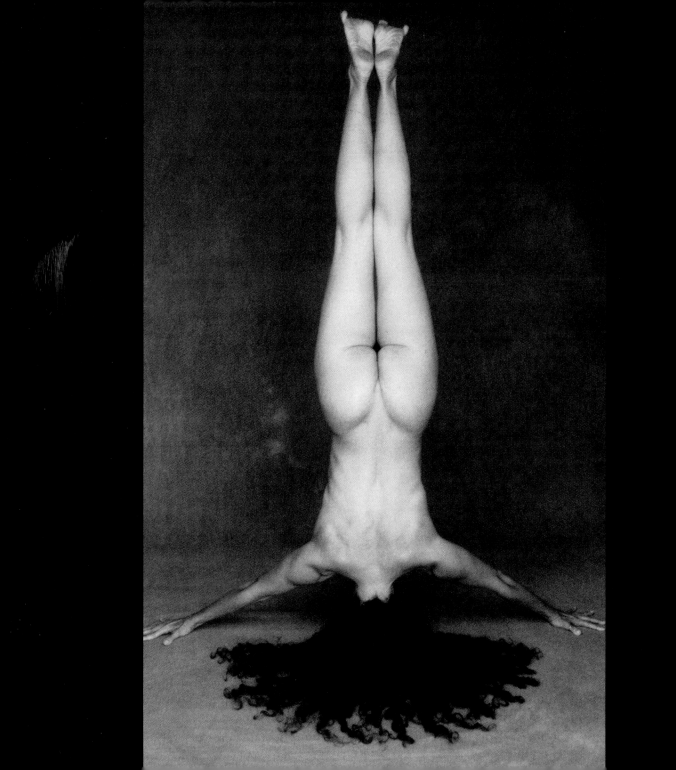

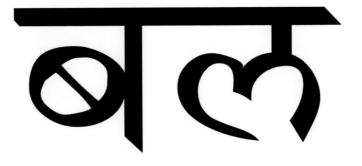

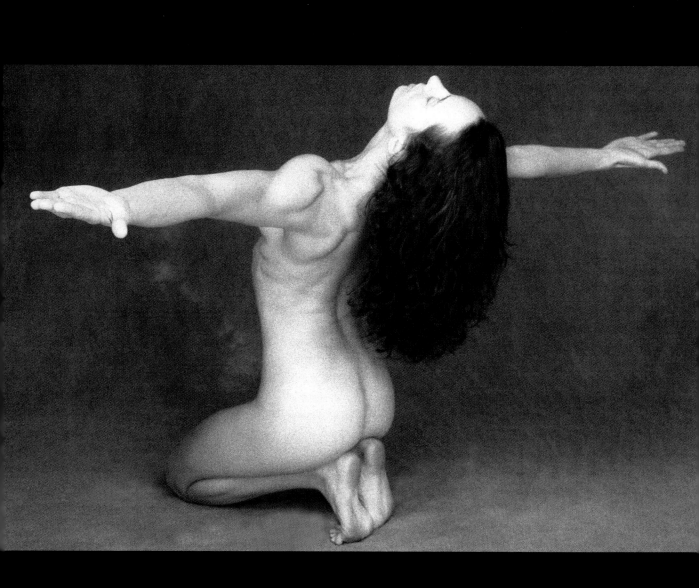

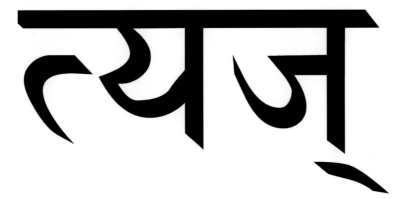

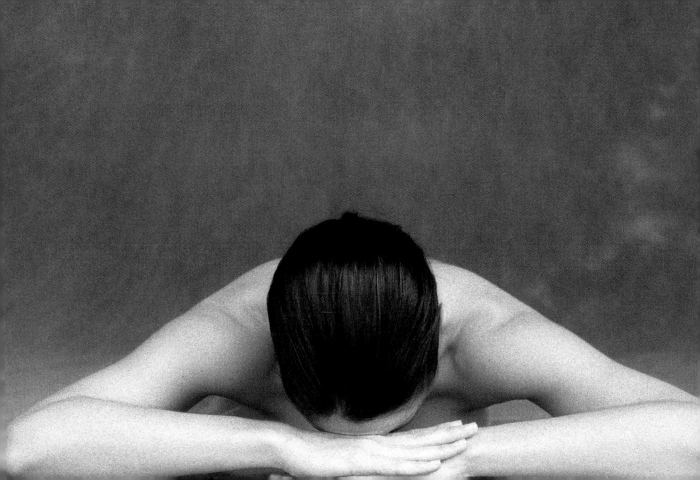

शम

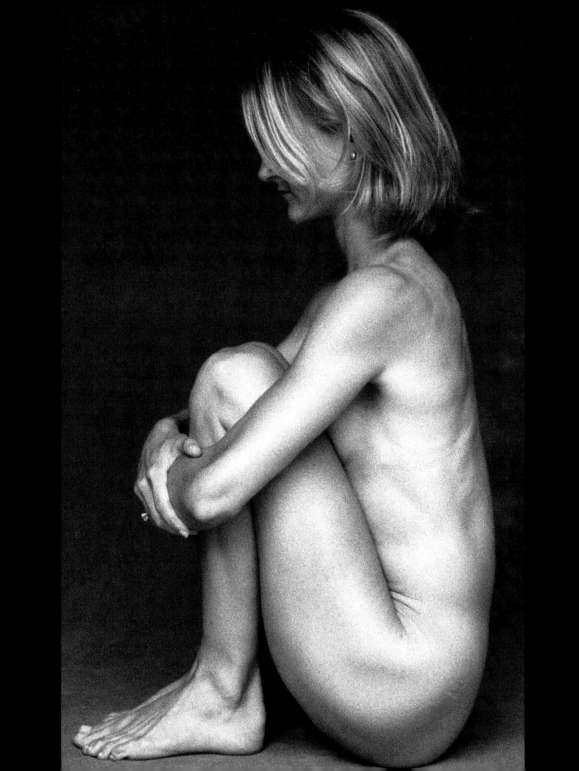

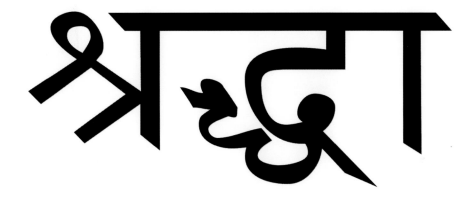

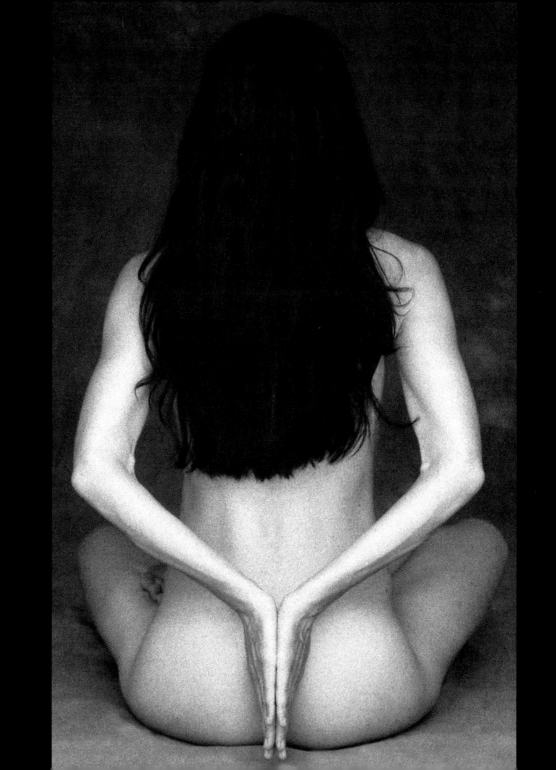

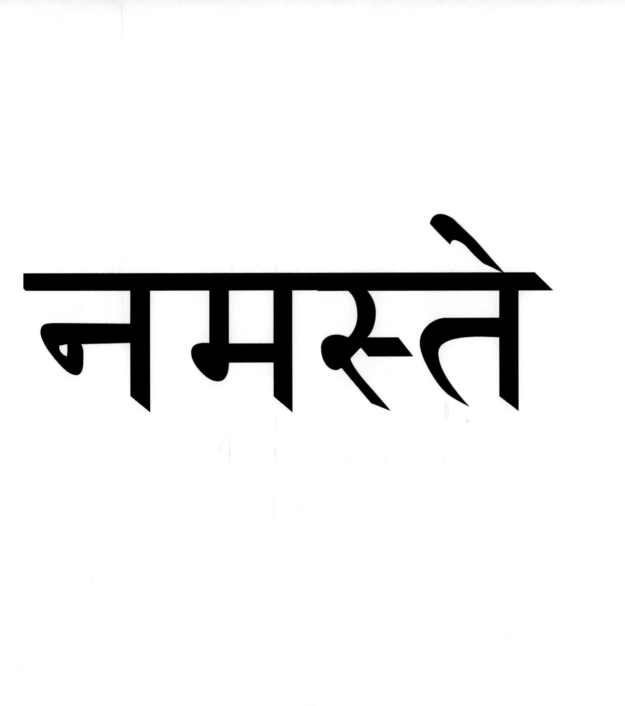

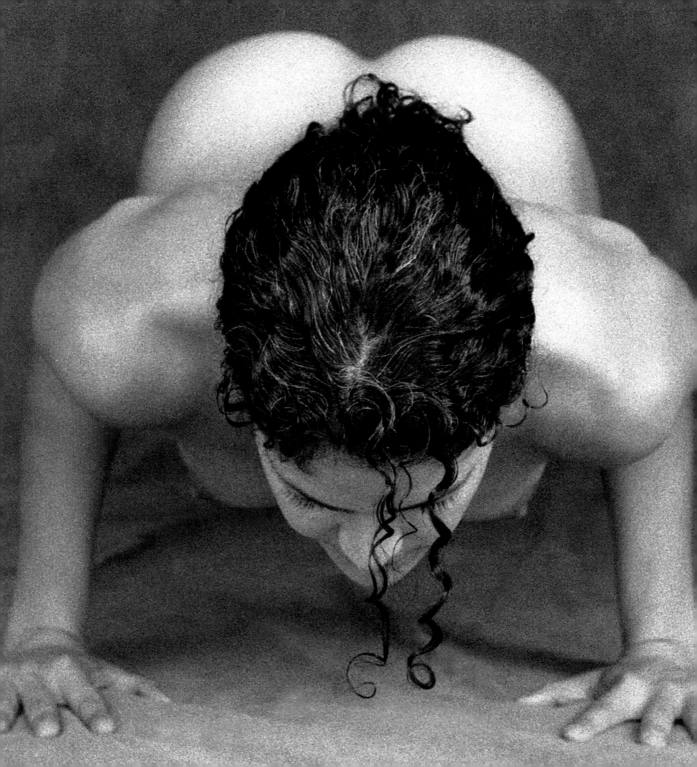

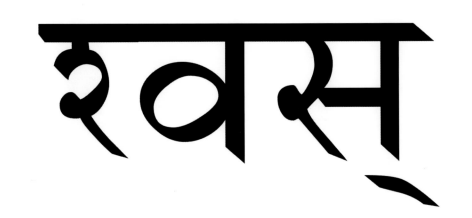

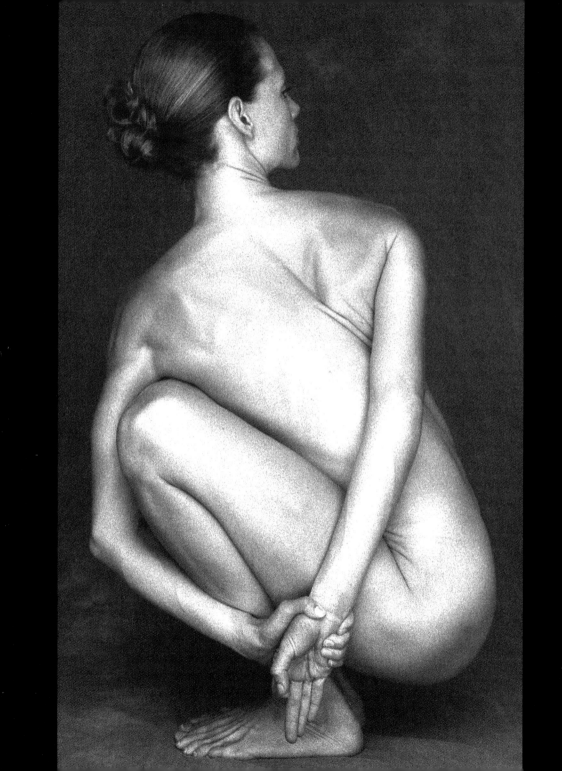

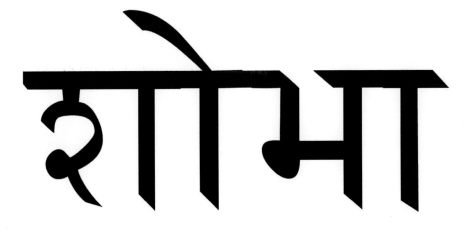

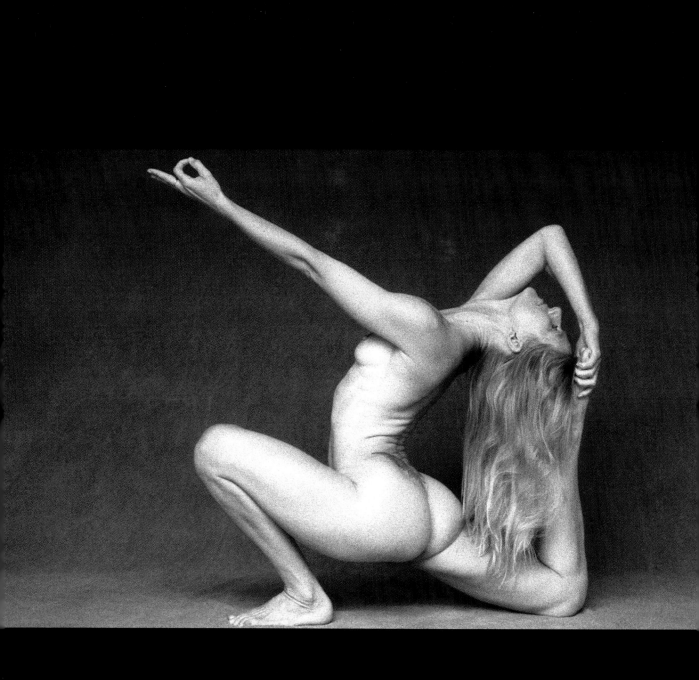

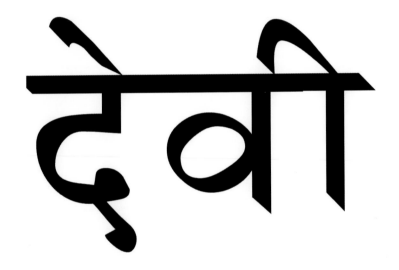

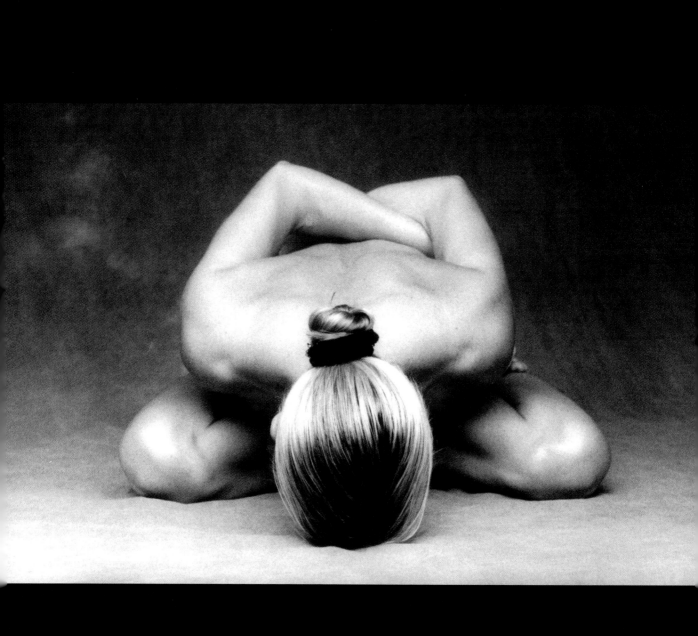

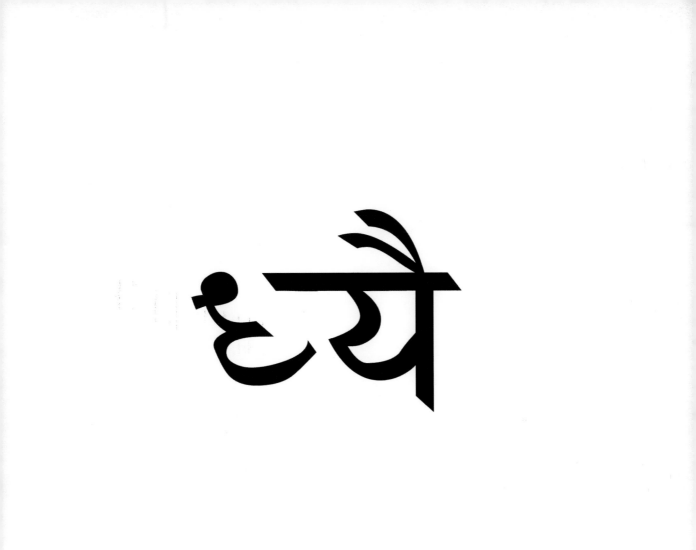

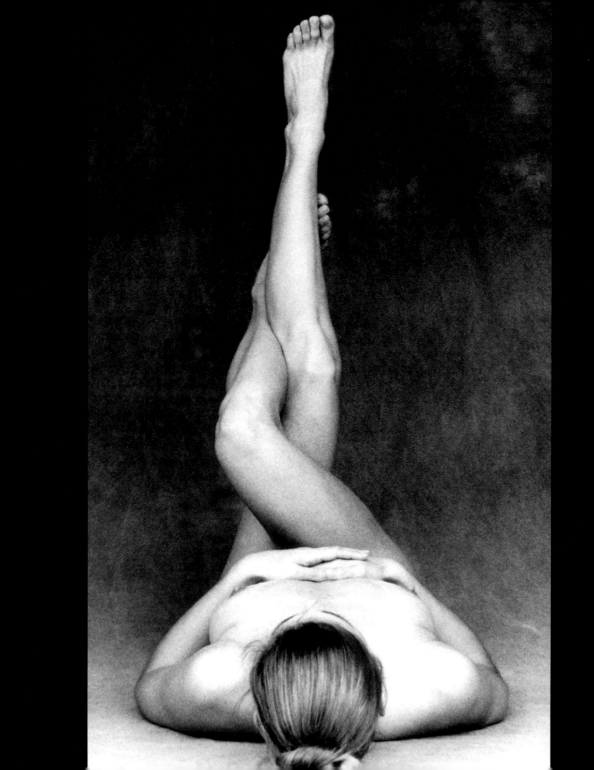

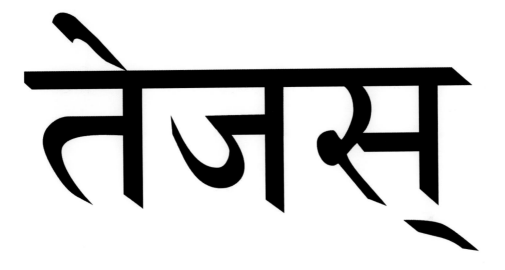

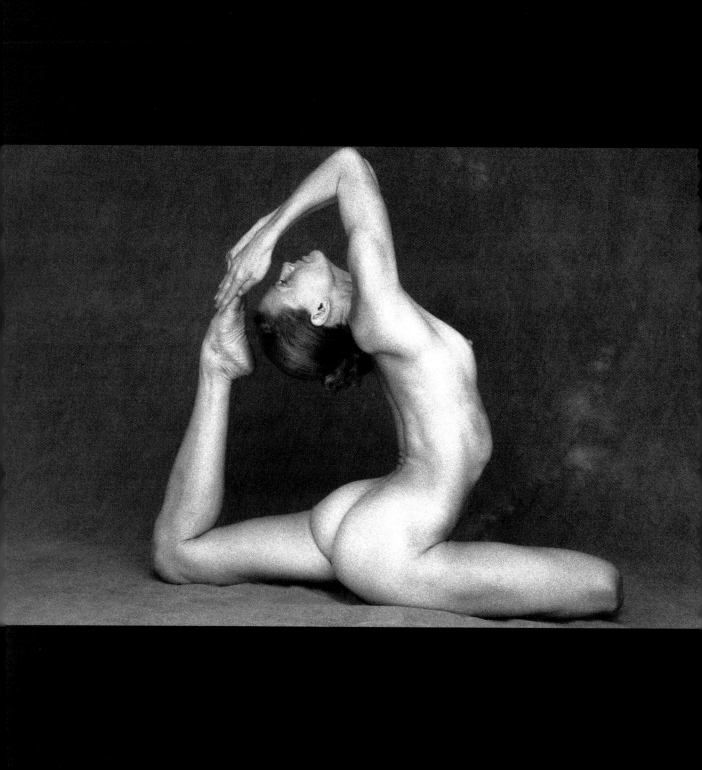

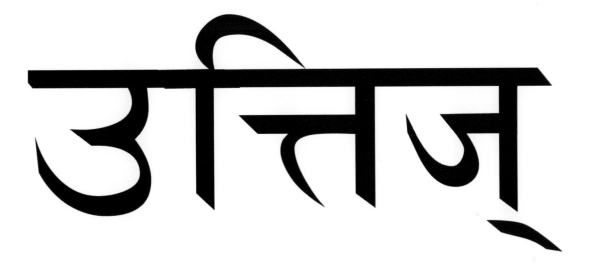

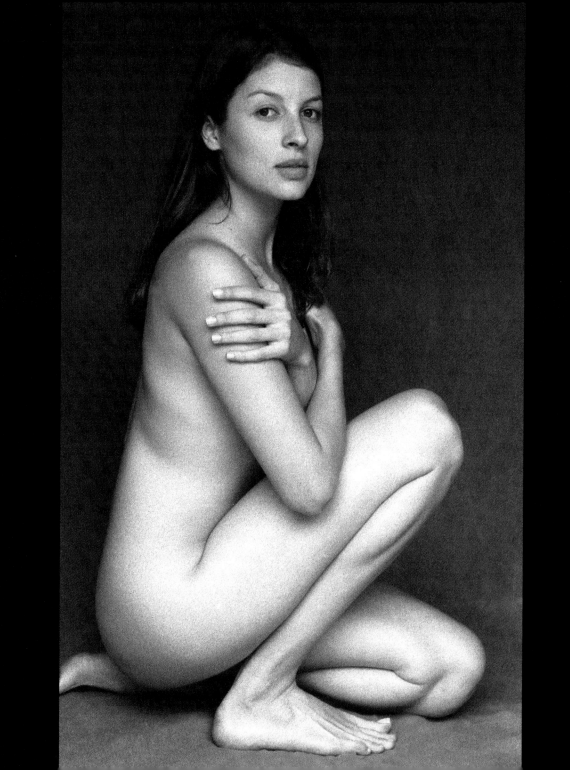

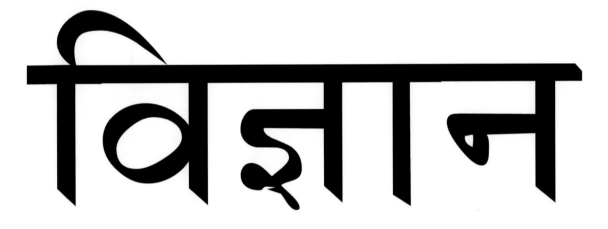

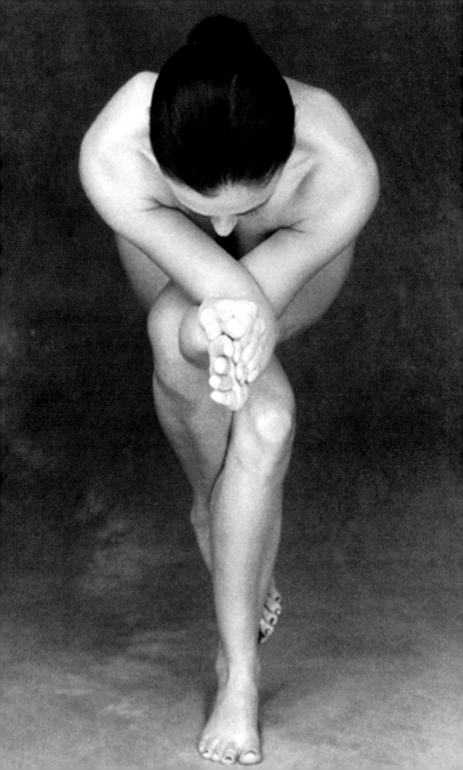

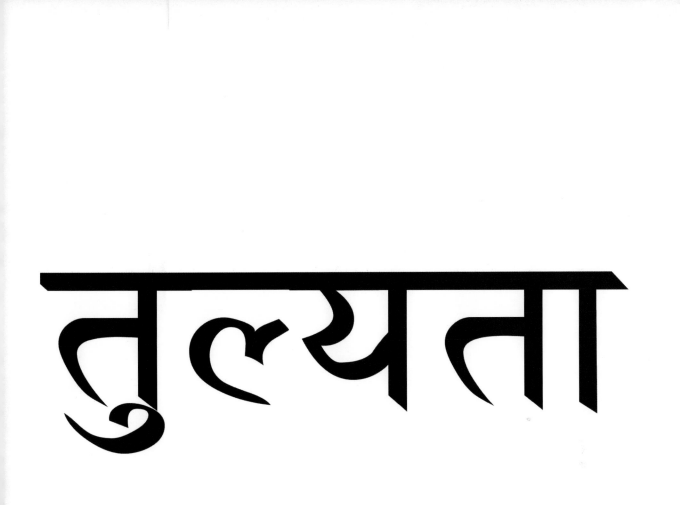

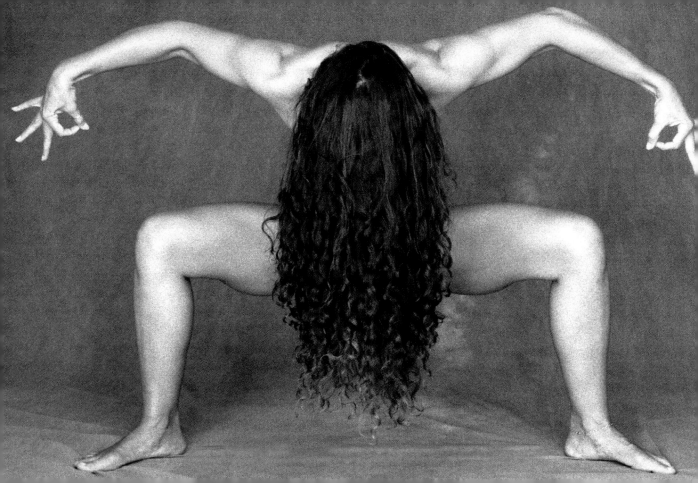

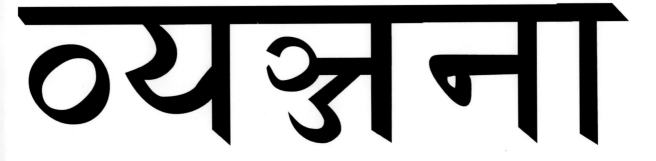

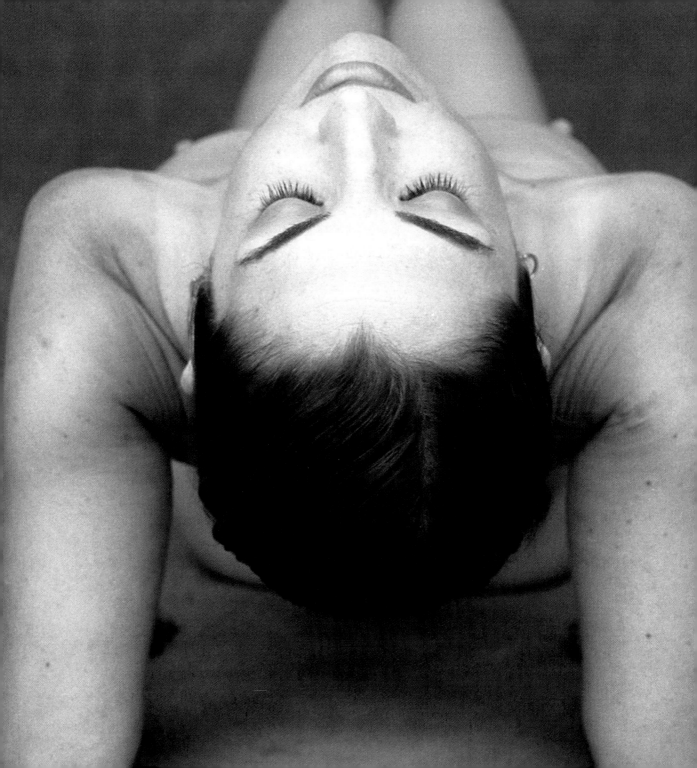

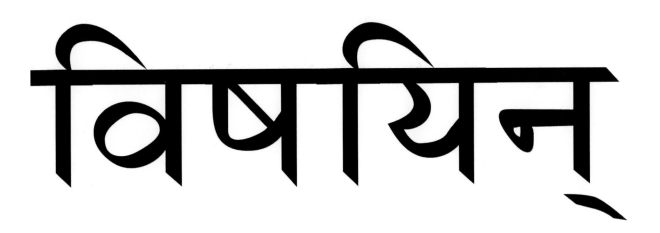

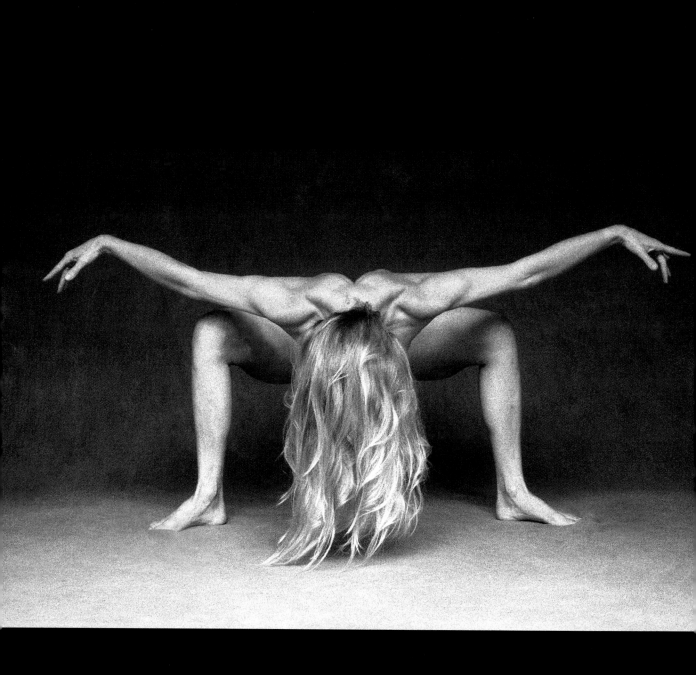

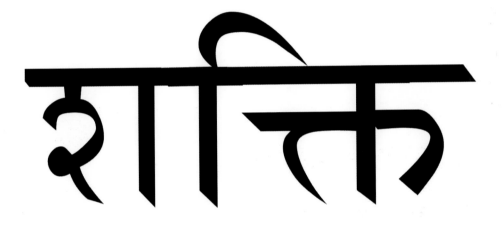

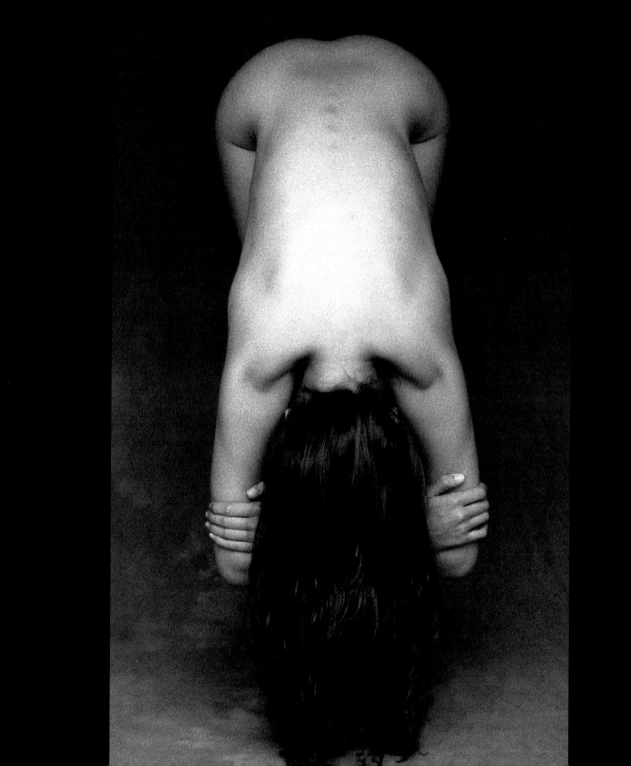

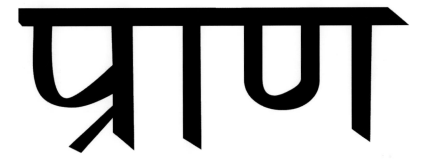

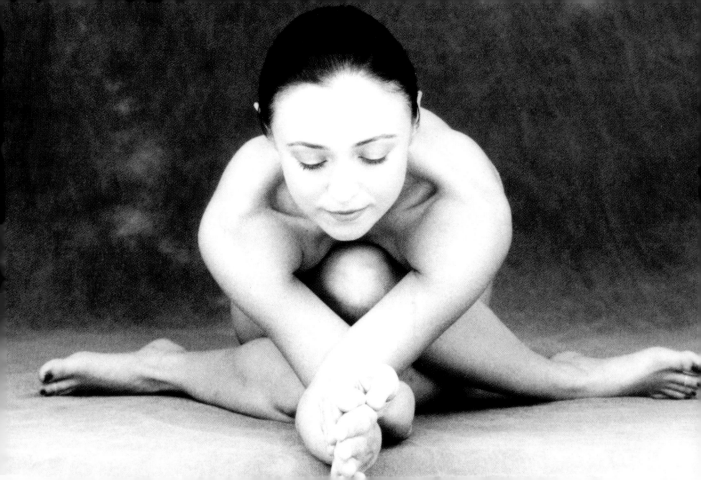

प्रज्ञा

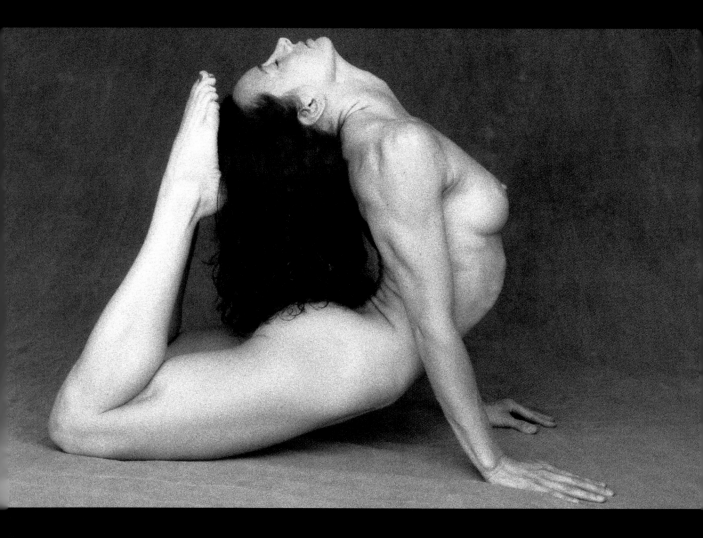

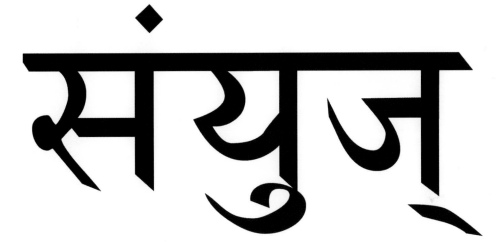

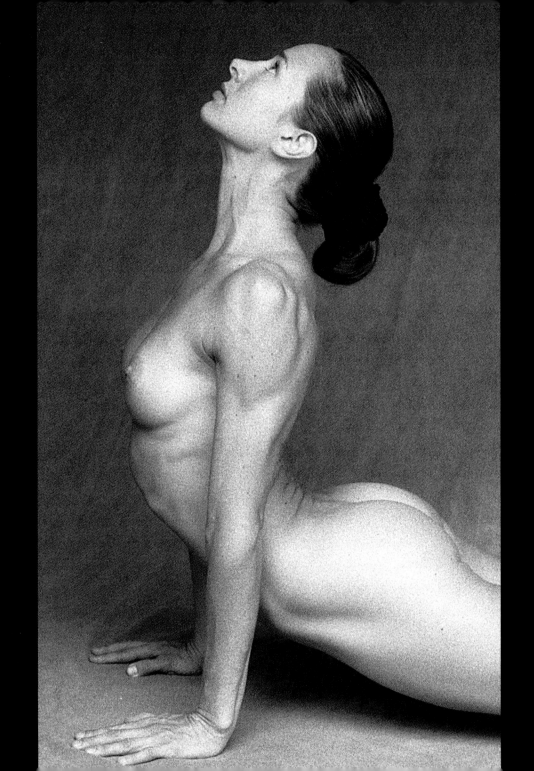

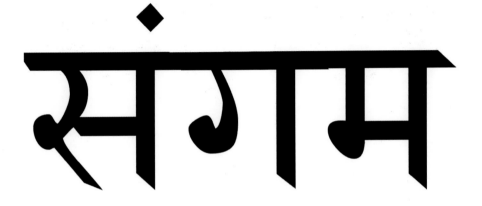

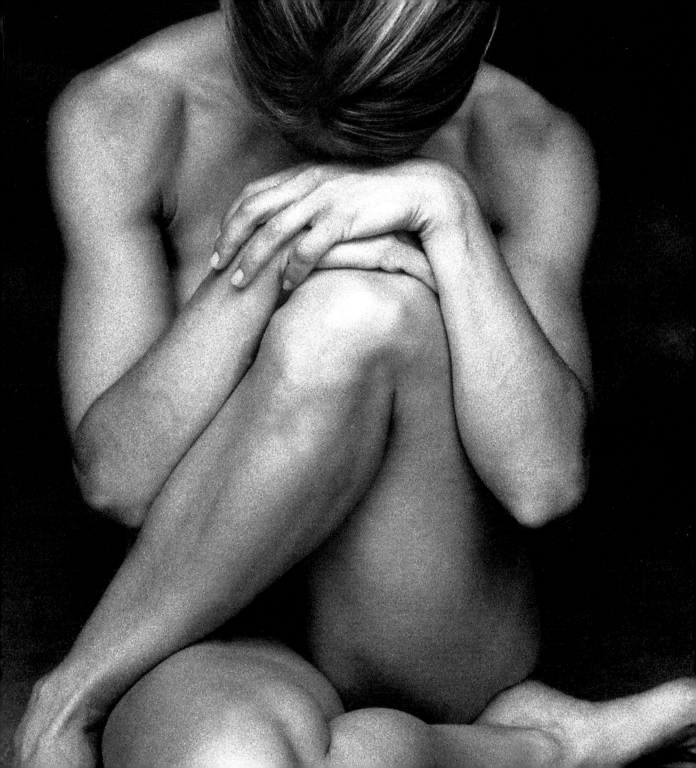

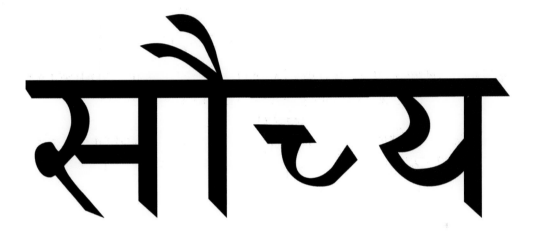

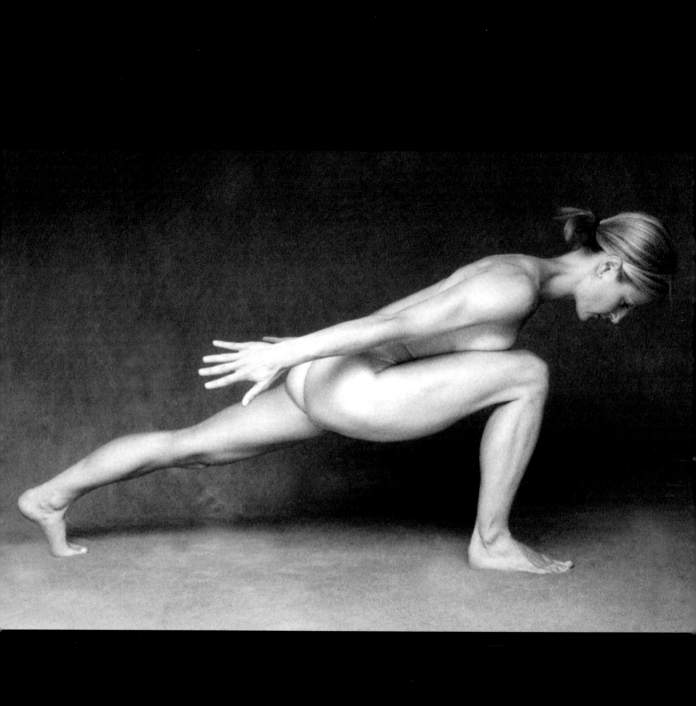

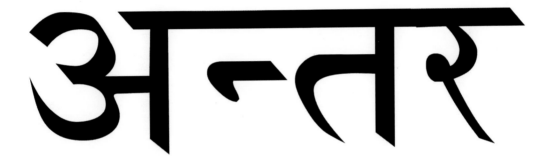

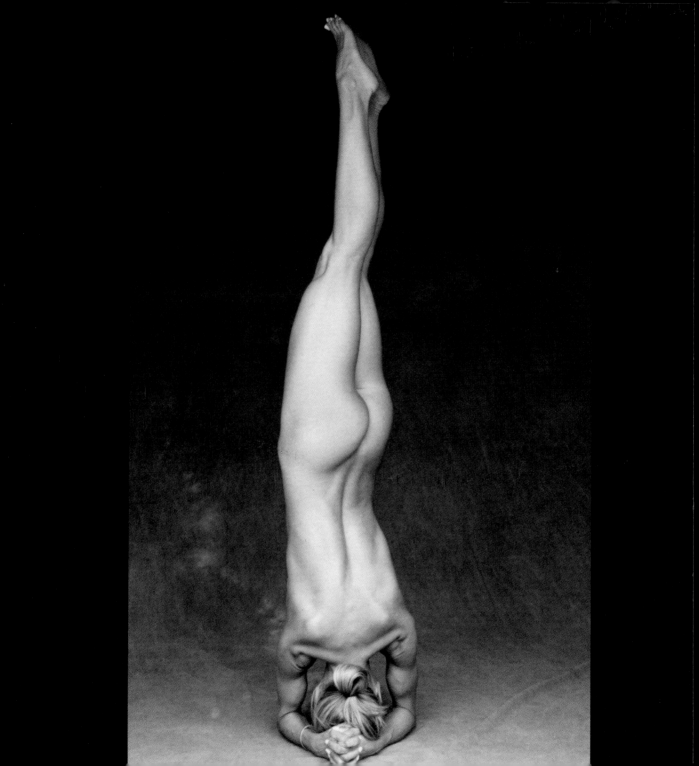

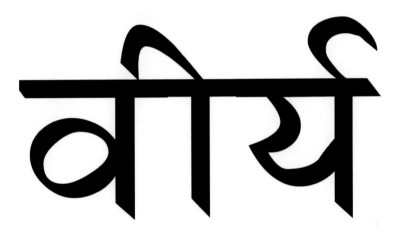

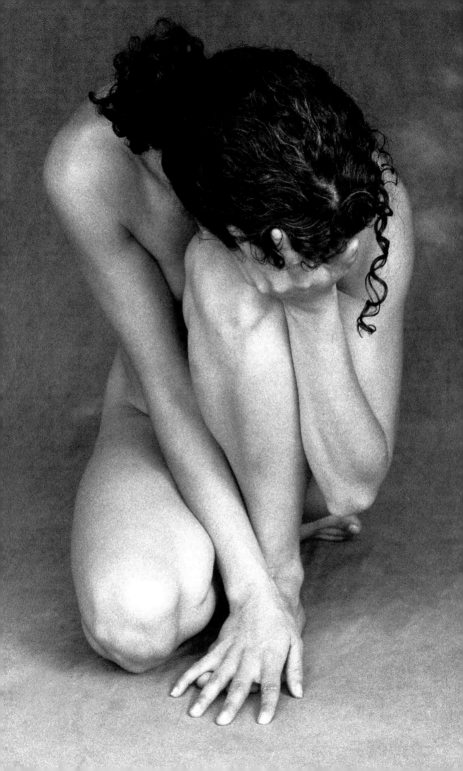

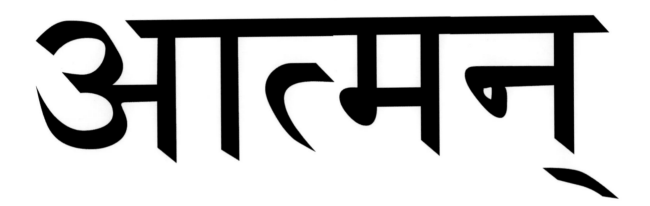

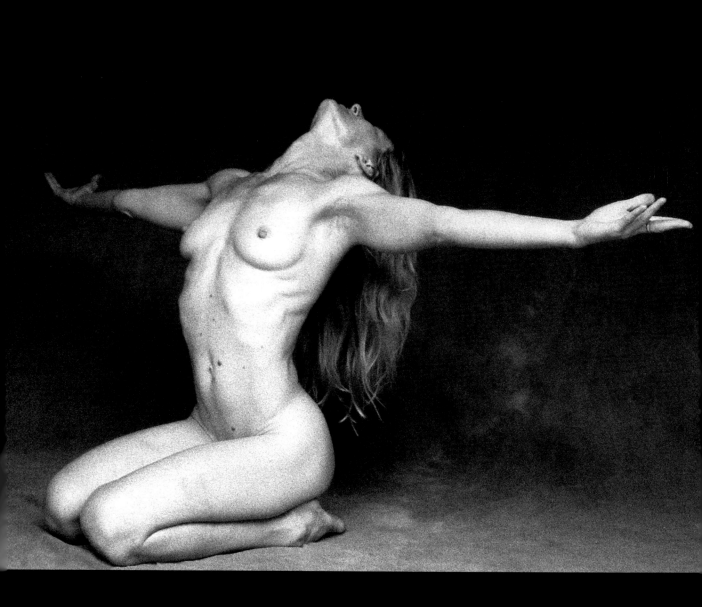

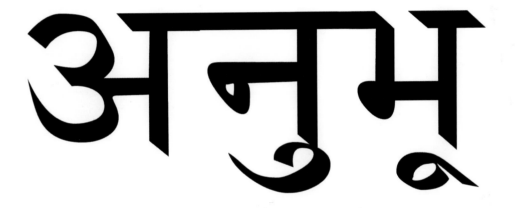

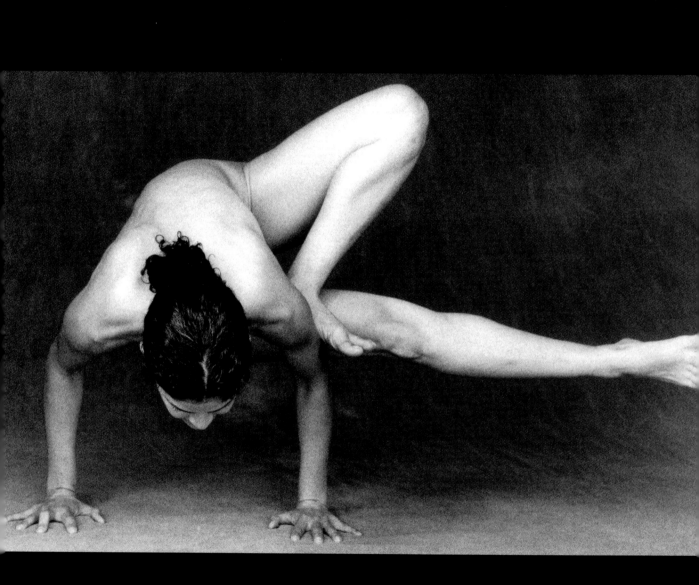

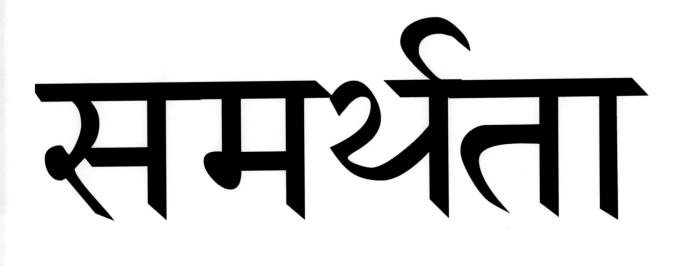

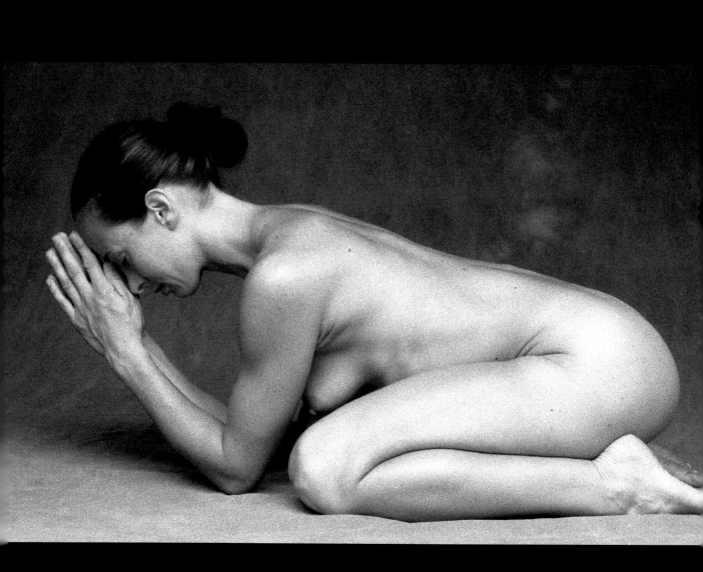

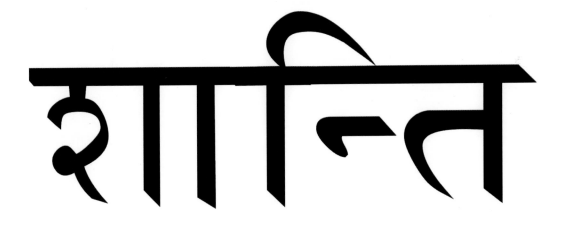

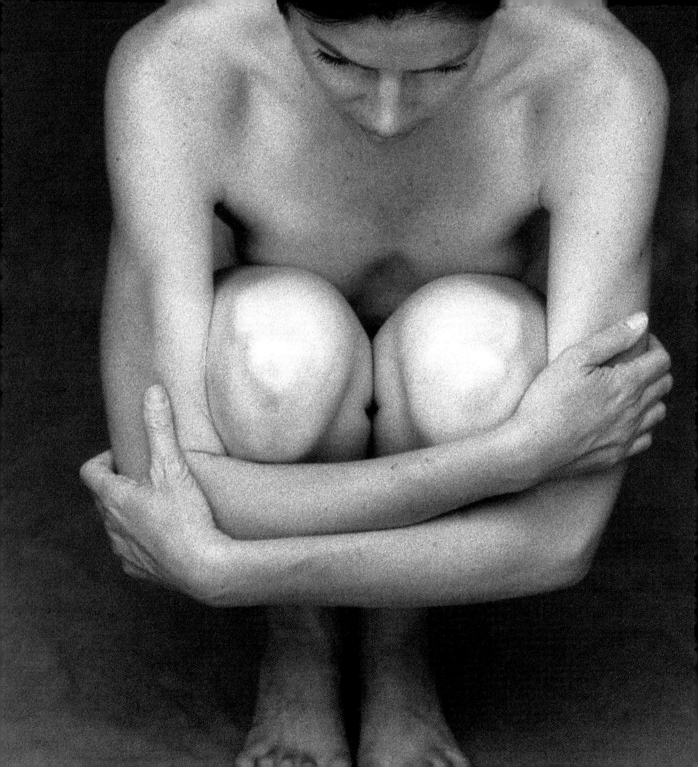

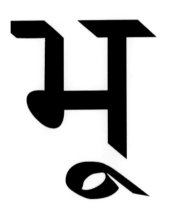

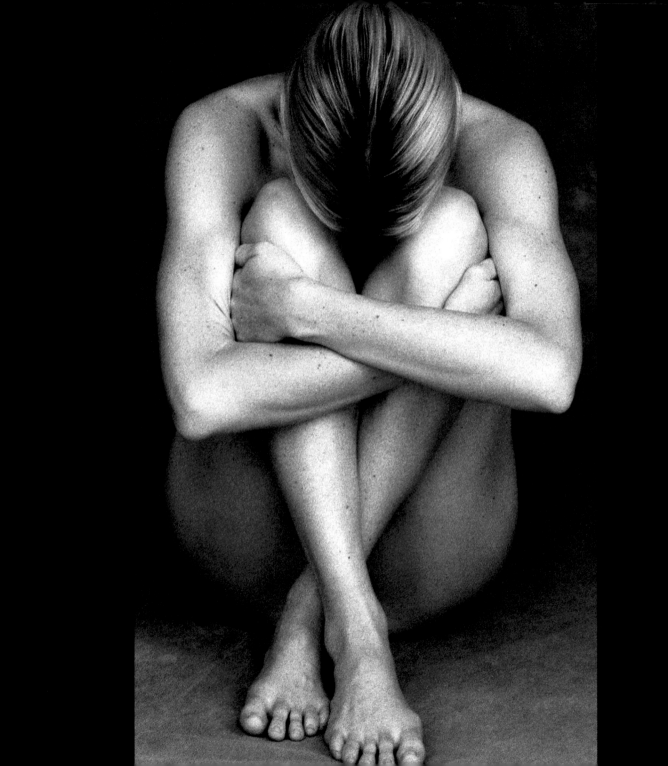

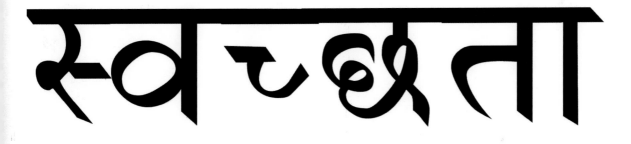

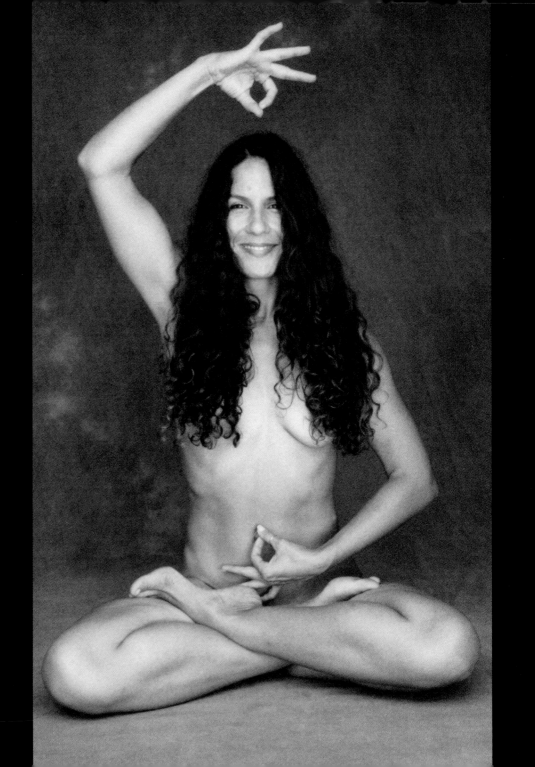

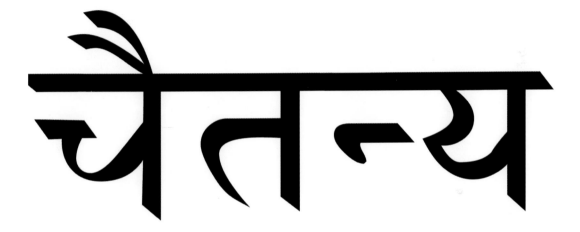

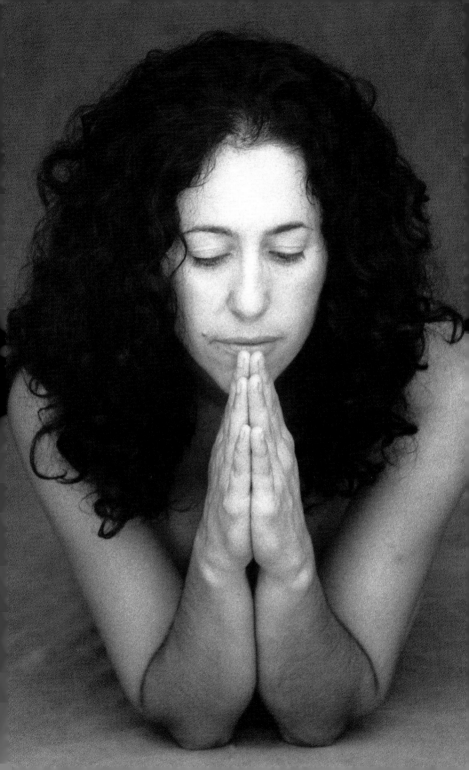

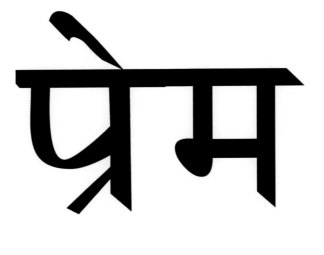

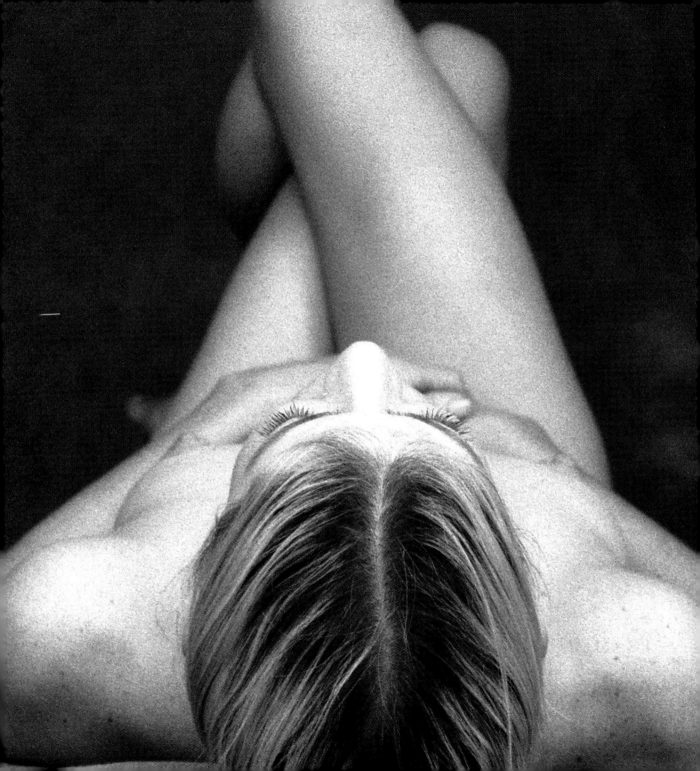

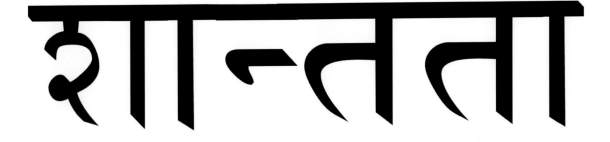

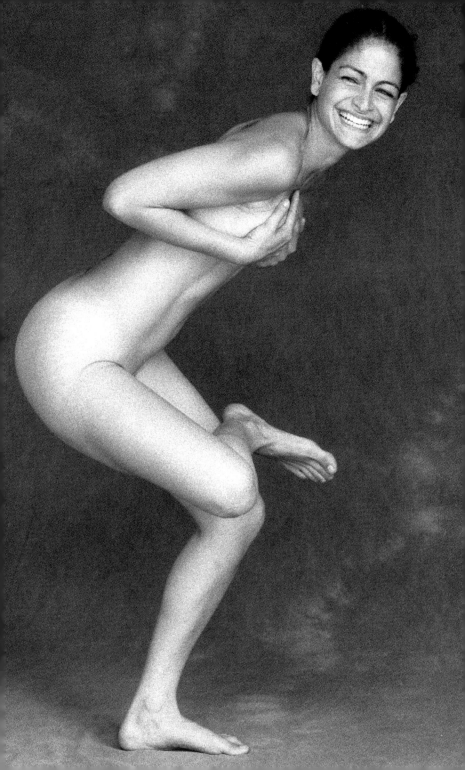

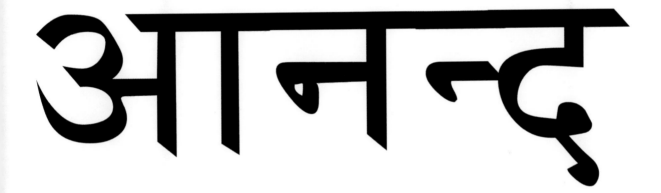

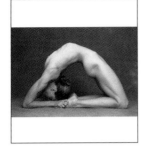

awake

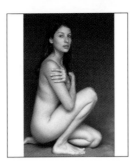

awareness

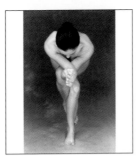

balance

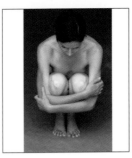

be

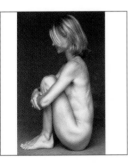

believe

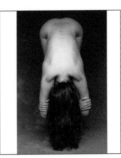

breath

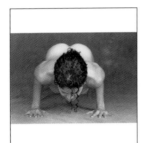

breathe

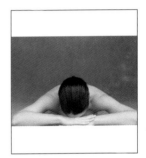

calm

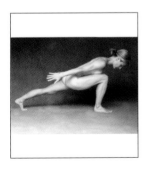

center

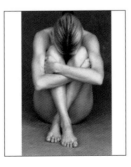

clarity

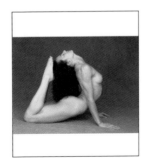

connect

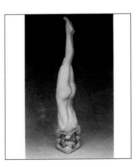

energy

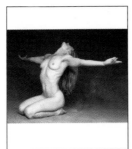
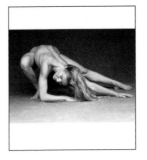
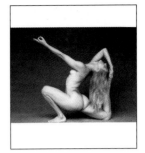
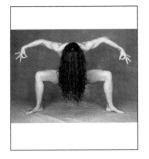

expression   feel   flow   goddess

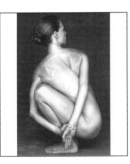
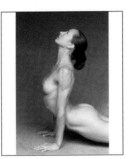
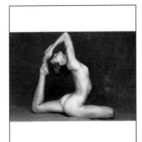
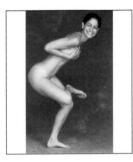

grace   harmony   inspire   joy

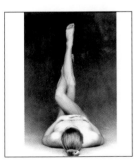
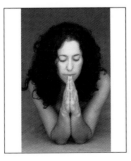
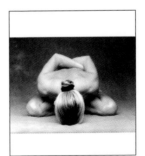
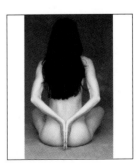

light   love   meditate   namaste

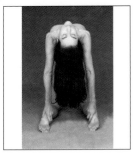

open

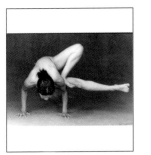

peace

power

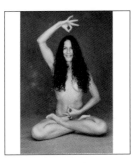

pure

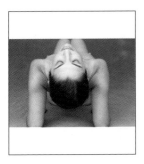

sensual

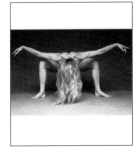

shakti

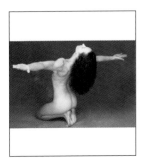

soul

spirit

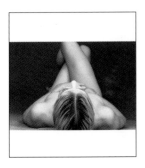

stillness

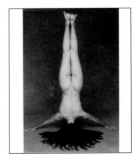

strength

surrender

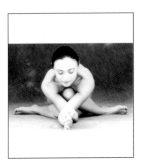

wisdom

Published by Davis Designs, Malibu, California.
www.victoriaphotography.com

Book designed by Amy Feldmann.
Photographs by Victoria Davis.

Printed in the USA.

ISBN 0-9715581-1-6

10 9 8 7 6 5 4 3 2 1